YOUR WEIGHT LOSS MASTERPLAN

*The Strategic Playbook for Root Cause Weight Loss
— No More Diets, Just the Moves That Work*

by

DR. JENNIFER R. WELCH

Founder of Root Cause Rewire^{TM}

For permissions or bulk orders, contact:

hello@RootCauseRewire.com

Book design and formatting by JRW Holdings, LLC

Printed in the United States of America.

First Edition: 2025

ISBN: 979-8-9992813-0-2

Cover design by JRW Holdings, LLC

This book is not intended to provide medical advice or replace personalized care. Always consult with a qualified health professional before making any changes to your wellness regimen.

THIS BOOK IS MORE THAN A MASTERPLAN — IT'S PART OF A MISSION
ONE ROOTED IN BOTH PERSONAL TRUTH AND A GREATER PURPOSE.

Growing up, Dr. Welch remembers standing in line with her mom at the local food pantry — picking up government cheese and powdered milk to help make ends meet.

In those moments, food was survival.
But in the quiet... in the overwhelm... and in the heartbreak that followed...
food also became comfort.

That emotional contradiction — the way food can both nourish and numb — became the root of a lifelong passion:

To understand.
To heal.
To help others break free from that same cycle.

This book is a complete strategic masterplan for weight loss — backed by science, shaped by personal experience — created to help you reset your body, rewire your patterns, and reclaim your power from the inside out.

And because Dr. Welch believes basic nourishment should never be a privilege, **a portion of proceeds from her programs support Feeding America®,** providing meals to families facing food insecurity.

Your transformation helps feed others.
Your healing becomes part of someone else's hope.

THIS BOOK IS DEDICATED:

To my mother, who always struggled with her weight and deeper self-worth.

To my patients, who make me push harder every day to be an even better provider and have often said I need to write a book.

To my family, who puts up with getting my leftover time but loves me anyway.

To my readers, who may have never understood why, despite all their efforts, their weight won't budge or maintain—this is for you. You were never broken. You just needed the right playbook.

To my future me, who will hopefully look back on her career and remember all the people she helped, making it all worth it.

CONTENTS

The "CMA" Disclaimer:

This book provides information for educational purposes only. It's important to consult with a doctor before making significant diet or lifestyle changes, especially if you have any underlying health concerns.

Using the suggestions in this book on your own in no way makes you a client of Dr. Welch, her companies, or her associates.

HAVE YOU TRIED EVERYTHING?

*"You may have made a few good moves...
but something still keeps knocking you off
track. You've got some of the right
strategies — but not the full playbook."*

You stare in the mirror, a familiar knot of frustration tightening in your gut. The latest plan—the one with the guaranteed results—hasn't delivered.

Maybe it even made things worse.

You're surrounded by weight loss solutions—books, programs, social media feeds—
yet lasting change feels just out of reach.

This isn't your fault.

You've been handed all the wrong playbooks.

The truth is, the weight loss industry thrives on quick fixes and surface-level answers.

One week it's keto. The next it's a shot, a shake, or a 75-day challenge.

But none of these address the **real, foundational drivers** of weight gain—like **inflammation, emotional triggers, hidden stress patterns, and toxic overload.**

It's like being dropped into a chess match with no strategy, no map of how the pieces move—and still being expected to win.

To succeed, you need to see the full board.
You need a plan that understands how your biology, brain, and behavior work together.

You need to stop playing defense with your health—and start leading.

This book is different.

If you have the **MINDSET** that true health starts from the inside out…
If you have the **MISSION** to live longer, stronger, and more freely…
This gives you the **MOVES** to make that mission a reality.

This isn't another diet.

It's a masterplan:

A strategic, science-backed reset that helps you understand your body's signals, repair your metabolism, and restore trust in yourself.

It's built on the Root Cause Rewire™ approach—a simple but powerful framework that helps you address your body's 3 core disruptors: **Sensitivities, Toxins, and Stress.**

These are the hidden forces that quietly sabotage your efforts—until now.

You'll uncover what's been holding you back, and finally learn how to **reset, reclaim, and rewire** your path forward.

This isn't a game. But it is a battle. And you deserve better than marching into it unprepared.

If you're ready to stop reacting and start leading your health with confidence...

Let's begin.

PLAY #1: RESET THE BOARD

Before you can make strategic moves, you must understand the landscape—and clear the board of hidden threats. Inflammation is the silent saboteur that distorts every system. If you don't address this, no strategy will stick.

Put Out The Fire Of Inflammation

Before you make your first move in any game, you must understand the board. In the game of weight loss—and more importantly, health—the board isn't just your body. It's what's already in play: hidden triggers, unseen threats, and chronic patterns. The most disruptive of these is inflammation.

Inflammation 101:

When you hear the word "inflammation", what comes to mind?

Inflammation literally means "in flames" or "on fire". Some cell (or more likely a whole bunch of cells), somewhere in the body, is "on fire." Inflammation is a complicated but natural response by the immune system of the body to fight off invaders, repair, and heal.

An acute inflammatory response is like a controlled fire—it helps the body heal after an injury. Like when you sprain your ankle and it gets warm and swells. This inflammation stays localized or limited to the injury area.

But when the flames never go out, the fire becomes dangerous.

Chronic inflammation is like an out-of-control fire—it's been going on longer and now doesn't stay in one space. This "fire" spreads and damages healthy tissues and is considered a root cause of many health conditions that are the top causes of death:

Heart disease, cancer, diabetes… But really, almost *any* chronic disease can be traced to inflammation.

And while conventional medicine has finally begun to recognize inflammation as a key player in disease, it still stops short of the more important question:

"What sparked the fire in the first place?"

That's like saying a house was lost to a fire without investigating *why* it started—was it faulty wiring, an unattended candle, or something else entirely? Without understanding the cause, the cycle just repeats.

Modern healthcare too often skips this root-level inquiry, opting to treat the symptoms of inflammation rather than preventing it at the source. But if you want to master your weight loss strategy—and protect your long-term health—you can't just chase symptoms. You have to stop the spark.

So, what causes the spark?

That's where things get interesting. Because inflammation, in and of itself, is not the enemy—it's a *natural* and *protective* response to injury or imbalance.

The real question we need to ask is: Why did the body feel the need to respond that way in the first place?

That's the question we'll begin to answer now.

What Causes Chronic Inflammation?

Inflammation isn't inherently bad—it's your body's natural defense against injury or illness. But when that response becomes constant, it shifts from helpful to harmful. Hidden sources of chronic inflammation include:

Processed foods, excess sugar, and unhealthy fats

Food sensitivities or gut imbalances

Toxins from your environment or personal care products

Poor sleep and chronic stress

Inactivity or even overtraining

Underlying infections or autoimmune issues

It's not about blaming your body—it's about learning what's been keeping it in fight-or-flight mode so you can shift back into healing.

What Does This Have To Do With Weight Loss?

If your house was on fire and you couldn't just run away, what would you do? Most likely, you'd get water and try to put it out, or if that wasn't appropriate, you'd use something to either smother it out or cut off its fuel supply.

The body is no different.

When your internal systems sense danger, the body acts swiftly. If your "house" (your body) is inflamed, you can't flee the fire, so the body does what it can to protect you:

- It holds on to water—like a firefighter trying to douse the flames.

- It builds up fat—as a barrier to shield healthy cells from further harm.

In short, inflammation makes weight loss *harder*.

And the longer it burns, the more systems it affects. Hormones. Brain chemistry. Sleep. Energy. Mood. This is why weight gain—or weight loss resistance—isn't just about calories. It isn't about "controlling" hunger....

It's about **calm vs. chaos** inside the body.

♟ Strategic Move #1: Cool the Fire, Control the Game

In the coming chapters, we'll explore the common culprits that keep this internal fire smoldering. But first, you need to recognize the signs of inflammation in your own body.

While medications like anti-inflammatories, antihistamines, or even weight-loss injectables like GLP-1s may temporarily dial down the body's fire alarm, they often do so without ever removing the actual spark. These interventions may modulate symptoms or suppress responses—but if the root cause is still smoldering beneath the surface, the game is far from over.

To truly win this match, we need to go beyond silencing the alarm and find out *why it was going off in the first place.* That's what the Root Cause Rewire is all about—addressing the hidden triggers that fuel inflammation, stress responses, and stubborn weight gain from the inside out.

Did you know?

While inflammation is involved in many health conditions, remember, it's a *normal* response to your body's threats.

In medical terms, the ending "-itis" literally means inflammation.

The start of the word identifies (in Latin roots) *where* the inflammation is located but it does not identify *why* the inflammation is there.

For example:

Condition	Latin Root	Meaning
Arthritis	*arthro-* (joint)	Joint inflammation
Gastritis	*gastro-* (stomach)	Stomach inflammation
Dermatitis	*derma* (skin)	Skin inflammation
Sinusitis	*sinus*	Sinus inflammation
Bronchitis	*bronchi*	Lung inflammation
Tonsillitis	*tonsils*	Tonsil inflammation
Conjunctivitis aka "pink eye"	*conjunctiva* (part of the eye)	Eye inflammation

Again, the word refers to the <u>where</u>, not the <u>why</u>...

Find the spark, reset the board.

SELF-CHECK: ARE YOU PLAYING WITH FIRE?

Acute signs (like a sprained ankle)
- o Pain
- o Redness
- o Swelling
- o Decreased function/movement

Chronic signs (long-term inflammation)
- o Fatigue or low energy
- o Skin problems
- o Joint pain and stiffness
- o Sleep issues/Insomnia
- o Mood changes
- o Brain fog/memory
- o Hormone imbalances
- o Digestive issues
- o Puffy face or water retention
- o Stubborn weight issues
- o Diagnosed with pretty much any health condition
  - • Heart disease, High blood pressure, High cholesterol
  - • Diabetes, Cancer, Arthritis
  - • Autoimmune diseases…to numerous to list

PLAY #2: KNOW YOUR OPPONENT

*""Let food be thy medicine and medicine be
thy food." — Hippocrates
Yet somehow, this wisdom got lost in
translation…*

Food as a Trigger

Hippocrates, often called the "Father of Medicine" and the basis of the Hippocratic Oath that we all know medical doctors recite upon graduation, lived from about 460—370 B.C. That's over 2000 years ago! He had many perspectives on health that still foundationally apply today.

Two of my favorite quotes that are attributed to Hippocrates are "All Disease Begins in the Gut" and "Let Food Be Thy Medicine and Medicine Be Thy Food".

With that in mind, it completely drives me nuts when I work with someone to decrease overall inflammation, and their medical doctor tells them, "What you eat has little to do with your (insert essentially any chronic health condition)."

Did they forget about Hippocrates? Did they forget about all the articles over the past two decades that link most chronic conditions to inflammation?

Here's the truth:

Foods are the inflammation trigger you have the **most** control over.

Beyond the usual suspects

Most people realize that these are not "good" for them:

- Processed foods—Ever try to pronounce most items on the food label these days? Many foods are engineered to taste good and last long on a shelf in food science labs across the globe but add little to nothing nutritionally.

- Sugars—Recent statistics show we consume 17 teaspoons **per day** on average (which equals 85 grams of sugar or a bit over 1/3 cup). This is more than in the 1970s and **over twice as much** as the American Heart Association recommends. (And this statistic seems *too low* to me, looking at what most buy in the grocery stores or out and about these days…)

- Refined carbs—Carbs that have been stripped of their fiber, bran, germ (and therefore most nutrients), such as white flour, white rice, pasta, pastries, cakes, cookies, and cereals.

The body quickly converts refined carbs to sugar, and too much of any macro (fat, carb, or protein) is stored as fat.

But what if you've already reduced or eliminated these…and you're still struggling?

What If "Healthy" Foods Are Harming You?

This is where food *sensitivities* come in. These aren't allergies, but they can quietly sabotage your progress with:

- Bloating
- Brain fog
- Headaches
- Fatigue
- Stubborn weight
- Mood swings
- Skin issues

It can be so challenging to try to figure out what might be behind all of this on your own, or even with professional guidance.

That's why I am an advocate of sensitivity testing.

Sensitivities versus Allergies

Many people assume that if they don't have a food allergy, then food isn't the problem. But **food sensitivities are more subtle—and far more common.**

Allergies (Type I immune responses) involve IgE antibodies and cause immediate, sometimes dangerous reactions—like hives, throat swelling, or anaphylaxis. Common allergies are from peanuts or shellfish. These reactions are what allergists test for using **scratch testing or blood work.**

Here's where the confusion happens: many patients believe that if they've had either of those tests, they've been "fully checked" for food issues. But that's not the case.

Sensitivities fall into Types II–IV immune responses. These delayed reactions can take **hours**— or even **days**—to appear, and often show up as fatigue, brain fog, bloating, joint pain, phlegm, or skin issues without any obvious "allergic" reaction.

And here's the problem: these types of immune responses don't show up on standard allergy panels. Most conventional doctors and even allergists rarely look beyond IgE-mediated reactions.

As a result, **many people continue struggling with hidden triggers—often the true culprits behind the very symptoms they're actively seeking help for**. Instead of identifying the root cause, they're often given medications to manage symptoms while the underlying sensitivity continues unchecked.

Because this deeper testing falls outside the standard care model, it's often not covered by insurance—not because it's ineffective, but because it's not yet widely adopted by mainstream medicine. That doesn't make it any less valid. It simply means it's part of a growing movement in personalized, functional care focused on *finding the root cause—* not just managing symptoms.

Identifying Food Triggers: 3 Options

You really have three main ways to uncover your food triggers: tracking, trial and error, or testing.

Option 1: Tracking

Keep a detailed food and symptom journal for at least 30–60 days. For best results, you write down all your foods and beverages consumed every day, and you also track your symptoms—pains, fatigue, mood, bloating, gut irregularity, headaches… everything.

At the end of the month, you look at both sets of data for patterns.

Maybe you eat spaghetti every Saturday night, and you see that you look 3 months pregnant on Sunday afternoon, and your clothes didn't fit so well that day, or your knee pain is worse on Mondays. You cut out the spaghetti and those symptoms get better and then tackle another pattern you find.

Pros:

1. Low to no cost: you can use any method to track as long as it is easy to go back and reference for patterns (paper, smartphone, etc).

2. It can be helpful to find some triggers and doesn't necessarily involve big diet changes all at once.

Cons:

1. *Time*. While you may not have to eliminate as many items as you find patterns, it takes time to track consistently, time to analyze your results, and time to trial possible offending foods. What if you find the cause of your

belly bloat, but your headaches still remain—
Do you keep going?

2. ***Errors***. Nothing is without the possibility of
   errors (we're all human, right?) but tracking
   takes consistency and detail to really have the
   clues you need to get the best results.
   Forgetting to track is a common issue, as it
   can be tedious and tiring.

3. Many trigger possibilities. From my example,
   it is hard to identify what it was about the
   spaghetti that made the difference—was it the
   gluten in the pasta? The tomato? The garlic?
   The parmesan sprinkled on top? Or a
   combination of several things?

Option 2: Trial and Error

Long considered the "Gold Standard" in
identifying food sensitivities, the elimination and
reintroduction method relies on careful observation.

You begin by removing common trigger foods
for a defined period—typically 6 to 12 weeks—to
allow inflammation to calm and the gut to reset.
Then, you gradually reintroduce these foods one by
one, watching closely for any return of symptoms.

Common trigger foods often include:

- Gluten
- Dairy
- Eggs
- Nuts and seeds
- Beans and legumes
- Sugars

This method can be effective but requires diligence, planning, and some trial-and-error experimentation.

Pros:

1. Eliminates statistically high-risk offenders upfront, often producing **faster symptom relief** than slower tracking methods.

2. As you reintroduce foods, you may discover that **symptoms you didn't even know were related**—like joint stiffness, brain fog, or bloating—suddenly return.

Cons:

1. **Beyond the main food categories**, it's difficult to know what else may be affecting you—leading to guesswork.

2. You might **eliminate foods unnecessarily**, potentially restricting your diet more than needed.

3. You may also totally miss a major offender for you if it wasn't part of the initial elimination list.

4. **Subtle or delayed symptoms** are easy to overlook, leading to premature reintroduction or misinterpretation.

Option 3: Testing

As I said, I am an advocate of food testing. It's helped me with many clients who've tried everything and still feel stuck. If offers a shortcut to identifying culprits you might never otherwise guess.

Sadly, mainstream medicine overall still tends to dismiss this (for various reasons that could probably fill another book!) and only gives much consideration to the Type I reactions.

However, without testing, I would be struggling to help determine that perhaps, like other patients I've worked with that...

Maybe you shouldn't eat beef...

...like we've found by testing an executive for one of the large corporations in my area, who was initially in disbelief that beef was part of their weight (and pain) problem. But then they later told me (after doing a reintroduction as planned), "Whoa, I felt it SO much, I couldn't believe beef was making me feel that way before!"

Or maybe you shouldn't eat chicken...

...like another patient whose abdomen would get so firm or hard off and on and would have embarrassing bathroom experiences that they thought were "normal"... until that all went away when they removed all their positive foods but returned when they reintroduced chicken too soon.

Or maybe you shouldn't eat apples...

...like a weight loss patient we had that when I talked to her for her consultation, I noticed she had a noticeable rash all over her neck. When I asked her about it, she said, "No one can figure it out... I've been everywhere: dermatology, allergy, even to Mayo. No answers, I just "deal with it," but it is embarrassing when it flares, especially at work."

But her rash **went away** a few weeks into her weight loss program and then incidentally returned one day. By examining anything from her sensitivities results report that she may have recently restarted around that time, it was found some apple cider vinegar was in a new tea she had started drinking…and apples were on her reaction list.

Challenging the apple idea purposefully revealed that apples were, in fact, her trigger for the rash. (She did fantastic on the weight program as well, but her rash was also a long-standing concern for her, so she was thrilled someone finally found the root cause.)

Or maybe you shouldn't eat dill pickles…

…like my daughter, who doesn't have a weight problem but is still a case that I think about when someone asks me if food testing could help them.

When my daughter was just 5 years old, sometimes when I would tuck her into bed, she'd tell me, "Mommy, I have a headache…"

Like any parent, that concerned me. I wanted to help her. And like the stories above, when the "offenders" for any particular symptoms aren't obvious, testing for sensitivities has helped tremendously.

I had her tested. We got her results and shared them with everyone that cared for her. A few weeks later, she spent the night with her grandparents. The next night, "Mommy, I have a headache."

Hmm...she hadn't had them in a while.

What was different?

Well, Grandpa loves eating baby dills with the grandkids, and a quick call confirmed that he forgot that "dill" was on her "no" list.

Was her headache from a couple of small pickles? About a week later, I tested it. Gave her a dill pickle. The next night, another headache. It then seemed pretty clear that the culprit was the dill.

And I will never forget (though now that she's older, she wishes I would!), but when I told her that I thought dill was the problem (but cucumbers were OK), her response was, "OH NO, NOT DILL PICKLES, THEY ARE MY LOVE!"

I reassured her, like I do with my clients, that it most likely wasn't forever. Just long enough for her body to heal and "forget" that it had a problem with dill.

Understanding Testing Options

In my practice, I have used about every type of sensitivity test option as my practice and as testing options have evolved. They all have pros and cons, and while they are done in accredited or certified labs, I admit none are 100% accurate. (But to put that in perspective, ANY diagnostic test has some potential flaws.)

So, you might be asking, why test? I liken it to a road map. It gives us a starting point, a list of items to monitor more closely, perhaps additional items we might never have realized, and has been significantly helpful in addressing triggers.

With that disclosure out of the way, let's talk about these different testing options and perhaps give you some insight into why I have my preferences.

Comparing Testing Options

IgG testing

This testing is focused on a Type II reaction (out of the four sensitivity response types). IgG food sensitivity testing is probably the most common type of testing. It measures the presence of IgG antibodies in your blood. IgG antibodies are part of the immune system's response and can be elevated in response to various things, including food. Since the pandemic of 2020, many people have a greater awareness of IgG testing, as it was a method used to test for COVID.

Pros:

1. Availability—some online websites offer this testing and most providers that offer food testing are *likely* using a lab doing this method.

2. Affordability—panels are often limited to the most common culprits or maybe up to 250 items overall.

3. It is done either at home with a blood spot (finger prick) or requires a blood draw.

Cons:

1. May detect old or inactive reactions: High IgG levels **don't necessarily** mean you have an active immune response to that item since there's variation in individuals as to how fast they go away. Like COVID testing (which was an IgG test) you can still show an elevated IgG level long after your active issue subsides.

2. Risk of false positives: High IgG levels could therefore, be misleading and lead to "positive" findings to foods that are no longer actively causing inflammation. Therefore, removal of foods unnecessarily can occur.

3. Limited number of items tested compared to other methods.

4. The use of blood spot or full blood draw can be a deterrent for some who are nervous about needles.

Other testing strategies:

Several labs offer alternative sensitivity testing approaches beyond standard IgG panels. I've worked with many of these methods in the past, and patients sometimes bring results from other practitioners for review. While I no longer use these specific tests in my practice, they each represent unique methodologies worth briefly highlighting for awareness.

ALCAT / MRT / Elisa ACT

- **ALCAT and MRT** utilize variations of a testing strategy that measures changes in white blood cell reactivity after exposure to various antigens. This is typically done through centrifugation (a spin-based method) and analysis of cell volume or behavior.

- **ELISA/ACT**, developed by Dr. Russell Jaffe, MD, involves live cell analysis via microscopy to detect immune activation after exposure to specific antigens. If the observed immune response exceeds a defined threshold, the item is marked as reactive.

Potential Pros:

1. These approaches aim to capture immune reactivity beyond Type II (IgG) hypersensitivities, potentially addressing broader immune responses (Types III and IV).

2. They often test a wider variety of substances than standard IgG panels.

Considerations:

1. They generally require larger blood samples. ELISA/ACT, in particular, recommends a larger-gauge needle to preserve cellular integrity.

2. These tests may be considerably more expensive than other methods for testing.

3. As with many forms of immunological testing, inter-lab variability has been reported. In some

cases, split samples from the same individual have yielded differing results across different methodologies.

Note: This overview is intended for educational purposes and does not serve as an endorsement or critique of any specific laboratory. Individuals are encouraged to consult with their healthcare provider to determine the most appropriate strategy for their personal health goals

My current testing preference: Bio-Resonance

The latest method of testing we've been using in my practice over the past few years is still considered the "new kid on the block" at the time of this writing; so new it remains the most controversial.

Yet the results we've seen after conducting over **1,200 tests** in our office are hard to ignore.

Clients regularly tell me that this type of testing was *pivotal* in their ability to finally break through stubborn weight loss resistance. For many, it was the missing piece.

Like the CSI-style test, this method uses a simple **hair sample**. That sample is analyzed by a **high-tech** computerized system for your individual energy signature—your **bio-resonance**—and then compared against a wide panel of potential triggers.

Now, let's pause here: bio-resonance or "frequency-based" testing isn't New Age or imaginary. It's roots actually date back to Hippocrates over 2,000 years ago. Just because something is difficult to measure by conventional scientific tools doesn't mean it isn't real—or powerful.

Bio-resonance literally means **"life frequency"** or **"life vibration."** It's where **biology meets physics.** And while that might sound futuristic, this idea is already part of many accepted tools in medicine:

- **Music therapy** (sound = vibration),
- **Color therapy** (light wavelength = frequency),
- **Red light therapy** (light energy impacting biology) with much research recently validating and supporting.

It's not "fringe"—it's **the future of personalized health care.**

Pros:

1. It is totally non-invasive—no needles or finger pricking!

2. No age restrictions like blood testing – even small children can be tested.

3. Comprehensive testing for a large range of items: foods, non-foods, food additives, etc.

4. Very cost-effective, especially with consideration of the number of items tested. The lab I work with tests more items on it's lowest panel than you can get with any of the blood testing methods. You get more data for your dollar.

Cons:

1. Skepticism: As the latest technology is still emerging, it's not widely accepted, even within many functional health circles…yet.

2. Potential for imperfect accuracy: Like all tests, it's not flawless. But in my experience, cross-checking with other testing methods, it has shown comparable results and has high client satisfaction.

Bottom line? Knowledge is power.

Get the data. Even if it's imperfect, it's a **huge** leap forward in uncovering hidden causes into the preventable root causes behind your symptoms, inflammation, or weight loss resistance.

But—and this is a big one—**you need coaching** to interpret the results properly. I often meet clients who've had this type of test done online or elsewhere but were given no real *guidance* on how to apply it. Without a clear plan, even the best data can feel confusing or overwhelming.

Get the right test. Get the right guidance.

It can be life-changing.

♟ Your Strategic Move #2: Test Before You Move

Smart players scan the board before charging ahead. Testing reveals what foods and other hidden sensitivities are helping—or hurting—your progress.

If you're ready to take the guesswork out of identifying sensitivities and want the same trusted comprehensive test options and my customized reports we use with my clients....

Scan the code or visit: https://www.foods2lose.com

SELF-CHECK: COULD SENSITIVITY TESTING HELP YOU?

How many of these common sensitivity-related symptoms do you experience regularly?

Digestive
- ☐ Diarrhea
- ☐ Constipation
- ☐ Bloated or gas
- ☐ Belching or reflux
- ☐ Stomach pain

Weight
- ☐ Binge eating
- ☐ Cravings
- ☐ Compulsive eating
- ☐ Water retention/swelling
- ☐ Over or Under Weight

Emotions
- ☐ Mood swings
- ☐ Anxiety/fears
- ☐ Irritability/anger
- ☐ Depression/Apathy
- ☐ Aggressiveness
- ☐ Hyperactive or Restless

Eyes/Ears
- ☐ Itchiness eyes/ears
- ☐ Drainage eyes/ears
- ☐ Ringing in ears
- ☐ Watery eyes
- ☐ Dark circles under eyes

Nose/Mouth
- ☐ Stuffy or drippy nose
- ☐ Drainage/mucus
- ☐ Often clears throat
- ☐ Sinus problems
- ☐ Hay fever

Head
- ☐ Headaches
- ☐ Dizziness
- ☐ Faintness
- ☐ Insomnia
- ☐ Twitches
- ☐ Confusion
- ☐ Poor concentration
- ☐ Stuttering
- ☐ Learning difficulties

Joint/Muscle
- ☐ Joint or body pains
- ☐ Weakness
- ☐ Muscle aches
- ☐ Arthritis
- ☐ Stiffness

Skin
- ☐ Hives
- ☐ Acne
- ☐ Hair loss
- ☐ Flushing
- ☐ Eczema

Other Symptoms
- ☐ Numbness/tingling
- ☐ Irregular heartbeat
- ☐ Rapid heart beat
- ☐ Chest pains
- ☐ Frequent illness
- ☐ Urgent urination
- ☐ Genital itch
- ☐ Fatigue/feel drained

PLAY #3 DEFEND THE KING

"A strong defense protects the entire board."

We all encounter toxins in our daily lives. From environmental pollutants to residues in food, these unwanted substances can accumulate in the body and contribute to chronic inflammation—a natural immune response with very unnatural long-term consequences. One of those consequences? Stubborn weight loss resistance.

In this chapter, the **King represents your immune system**—your body's frontline defense against these toxic intruders. When the King is compromised, the whole board is at risk. This chapter explores the hidden impact of toxins and heavy metals on your health and weight journey— and how to fortify your body's natural defense system.

A Startling Legacy

Think you're safe from toxins? Think again. A landmark study by the Environmental Working Group (EWG) found an average of **200 industrial chemicals and pollutants in the umbilical cord**

blood of newborn babies in the U.S. Yes, exposure can begin *before* birth.

These substances have been linked to:

- Developmental problems
- Learning disabilities
- Increased risk of chronic disease

And that's just the beginning.

This legacy is not your fault—but it is your responsibility to address.

Heavy Metals: A Looming Threat

Heavy metals are metallic elements with high density that can be toxic even in small amounts. While they exist naturally in the environment, our modern exposure levels are far from natural. Some are stored in the bone marrow, quietly creating long-term stress without obvious symptoms. Others can reach the brain, interfering with mood, memory, or energy.

Common Sources of Heavy Metal Exposure

Heavy metals are truly everywhere in our world. Even with the best of intentions, you may be getting exposed to toxins from unexpected places. Here are some of the more common sources, but this is not a complete list:

- Food and Water
  - Larger fish (mercury – tuna, swordfish)
  - Rice and well water (arsenic)
  - Shellfish, organ meats (cadmium)
  - Old pipes or plumbing (lead)
  - Aluminum cookware, food additives (aluminum)
  - Even chocolate!
- Dental and Health
  - Silver (amalgam) fillings (mercury, nickel, tin)
  - Nickel crowns or braces
  - Certain antacids and vaccines (aluminum)
  - Contaminated teas and supplements (yes, even products meant to help may be a source, particularly as many come from regions with soil contamination)
- Lifestyle and Environment
  - Old pipes or private wells
  - Industrial zones or farm runoff
  - Jewelry (nickel)
  - Imported goods, toys, or paints
  - Cigarette and e-cigarette smoke or vapor (arsenic, cadmium, lead)

- Landscaping mulch and pressure-treated wood (arsenic)
- Military service – thank you Veterans, but I often find heavy metal burden affecting our service men and women
- Indoor dust and poor ventilation

Environmental Toxins: Beyond Heavy Metals

Other toxins silently steal nutrients and burden the body.

We encounter these various other toxins in everyday life, including:

- E-cigarettes and vaping – Often assumed safer than traditional smoking, these devices release aerosols containing ultrafine particles and metals like nickel, cadmium, and lead.
- Pesticides and herbicides: These chemicals used in agriculture can leave residues on produce and contribute to inflammation.
- BPA and phthalates: Found in plastics, these chemicals can disrupt hormones and potentially worsen inflammation.
- Household cleaners and personal care products: Some chemicals in these products

can irritate the skin and potentially contribute to systemic inflammation.

Health Effects of Heavy Metals & Toxins

Heavy metals and other toxins can disrupt various bodily functions and contribute to:

- Disrupt the immune system
- Impair energy production and cellular repair
- Contribute to mood swings, memory issues, and poor focus
- Create digestive problems and constipation
- Reduce bone density or mineral balance

One hidden pattern is that the body often **stores toxins in fat cells**, using them as safe-keeping until it's confident the release will be safe. This mechanism may be one of the biggest contributors to weight loss resistance.

Detoxification Support

While our bodies have natural detoxification processes, heavy or extended exposure to toxins can overwhelm the liver's ability to keep up.

In my functional practice, I often use mineral-based support to give the liver an assist in its normal job safely. I have found it to be helpful without much risk of harm (aside from detoxing too quickly, which those detox effects (called "Herxheimer" reactions— feels like a detox flu) usually go away within a few days if they do occur) to use specific minerals to "grab" onto heavy metals and assist the body's normal elimination process.

Sometimes the detox process is sluggish, so providing nutrients to assist the liver is also needed, and for that, I also can use vitamins and minerals to help the phases of detoxification done in the liver.

Some medications may impair liver and kidney detox pathways but you should NEVER make any medication changes without help from your medical provider.

Testing for Heavy Metals: What You Need To Know

Not all heavy metal tests are created equal. If you're concerned about toxin exposure, it's important to understand your options:

- **Blood tests** only detect recent or acute exposure. They can show what's circulating now but often **miss what's being stored** in tissues.

- **Urine provocation tests** (using a chelating agent) help identify what's mobilized from tissue, but results can vary depending on the chelator and the body's detox ability at that moment. The agent used can add stress to the kidneys if not done properly, so this method is not suitable for everyone and needs qualified supervision.

- **Hair mineral analysis** offers a **non-invasive snapshot** of chronic exposure, especially for metals like aluminum, mercury, arsenic, and lead. While not perfect, it can give clues about long-term patterns.

Many conventional practitioners may only offer blood tests, which—while useful in certain cases—can falsely reassure you that everything is "normal" even when deeper toxicity is present.

♟ **Pro tip:** If you're curious about options for testing for hidden toxicities, message my team at hello@RootCauseRewire.com with the subject: TOXIN TESTING for more options on ways to begin exploring your body's burden.

A Deeper Layer: What If There's Something Behind the Metals?

One fascinating and emerging idea is the role of **deuterium**, a naturally occurring isotope of hydrogen that's slightly heavier than the kind your cells use most efficiently. While small amounts are normal, **excess deuterium may interfere with mitochondrial function, reduce energy output, and slow the body's ability to detoxify.**

Some researchers suggest that **rebalance deuterium levels—and you may naturally rebalance metals as well.** That's because your mitochondria (the cell's energy centers) depend on clean water, sunlight, deep sleep, and metabolic rhythm—all things we're discussing in this book as essential to healing.

As of now, I am unaware of an available test to measure deuterium levels inside the body—but many of the **strategies for reducing toxic burden also support deuterium balance**: natural light exposure, movement, deep sleep, and staying well hydrated with clean, mineral-balanced water. While research is still unfolding, this reinforces a simple truth:

True detox isn't just about removing toxins—it's about restoring balance, energy, and flow.

If you're already addressing inflammation, food triggers, hydration, and movement, this deeper layer may be a future frontier in your health journey.

Final Thought: Your Body, Your Battlefield

You may not be able to eliminate every toxin—but every small step to reduce exposure gives your body more capacity to heal, shed excess weight, and function the way it was designed.

I often tell my clients: If you don't use a filter, you ARE the filter....

♟ Strategic Move #3: The Diagonal Detox

In chess, the bishop's strength lies in its long-range power—cutting across the board to clear obstacles that once seemed out of reach. Your body does its best to filter and adapt, but when the burden gets too heavy, metabolism stalls.

Dietary Choices:

- Choose organic produce, especially those on the EWG's Dirty Dozen list: https://www.ewg.org/

  ♟ Quick tip: If you eat the peel, organic is usually best.

- Avoid processed foods, full of chemicals for shelf stability; shop the perimeter of the grocery store where most fresh foods are located.

- Opt for low-mercury seafood like salmon or sardines

  o Bottom-dwelling seafood is a higher risk for toxins

Environmental Adjustments

- Use filtered water for drinking, cooking, and showering. Best is a whole-house system so all sources are covered in your home.

  In our area, it is amazing (or a little frightening) how fast our water filters need to be changed. Many of my patients have noticed real health improvements after paying attention to something we often take for granted... water.

  ♟ To find out what whole-house water filtration system we currently recommend, send an email to hello@RootCauseRewire.com, subject: WATER

- Improve indoor air quality with HEPA filters on your vacuums and ventilation systems.

- Read ingredient labels on personal care and cleaning products, opting for more natural ingredients when possible.

PLAY #4: TRAIN THE TROOPS

"Even the smallest pieces can shift the outcome of the game."

In chess, Pawns may seem insignificant—but when trained and moved strategically, they become game-changers. Likewise, your daily food decisions might appear small, but repeated over time, they shape your metabolic momentum.

This chapter is about training your portions—and your perception—to support sustainable weight loss without falling prey to the silent saboteur: portion distortion.

The Psychology of "More is More"

Our environment plays a huge role in how much we eat. Giant restaurant meals, oversized packaging, and "value" deals are visual cues that shift your perception of normal.

Research shows that when we're served more, we eat more—**even if we're not hungry.** This disconnect between hunger and portion size is one of the most powerful drivers of gradual weight gain.

It's not just what you eat—it's how much, how often, and how automatically.

Breaking the Cycle

Mindful Awareness

Mindful eating is your mental training ground. Savor each bite. Pause halfway. Check in with how you feel. Don't eat just because it's on the plate—eat because your body is asking for nourishment.

But let's be real. In a stress-filled, on-the-go life, mindfulness often takes a back seat. That's why many clients do better retraining with structure first—then layering mindfulness back in for long-term maintenance.

Measure to Rewire

I often ask: *"How much protein is a portion?"* Most people hold up a palm—fair start, but inconsistent. A standard portion of meat is about **4 ounces**, but visual estimations can be wildly off.

I recently bought a pack of chicken that had two large breasts. I took a photo of the package and started asking my clients how many servings they thought it offered.

Without hesitation, everyone said two. But those chicken breasts were large—it was a 20 oz package. The label said 5 servings. Clients instinctively assumed two pieces = two servings... not five. That's portion distortion in action.

Grab a food scale. For a few weeks, measure your proteins, starches, and fats. You'll quickly recalibrate what "enough" really looks like. You'll probably find yourself a bit surprised at the amount of food you **really** need to feel full and satisfied, especially when you eat nutrient-dense foods.

Hello hydration. One of the simplest, most overlooked tools for metabolism and detox is water. Slight dehydration can mimic hunger and bring on fatigue, slowing down your metabolism. People often overestimate how much they get in a day.

   A good rule of thumb is to drink half your body weight in ounces per day—often that is much more than the "8 glasses a day" idea...unless you weigh 128 pounds.

Don't exceed one gallon of water per day unless directed by your doctor. Overhydration can throw off your electrolytes. But also remember that ice takes up space in the cup, so it's best to measure. Get a pitcher and fill it with your target water amount for the day. Set a goal to drink that every day.

Harnessing the Power of Perception

Here's something few people realize: your brain doesn't just rely on hunger to tell you when to stop eating—it uses visual cues. When food looks abundant, your brain feels satisfied. When it looks scarce, it stays on alert.

That's where plate size comes in. Swap a large dinner plate for a smaller one, and the same amount of food appears more generous. Your brain registers "enough" sooner, which leads to less overeating—without any willpower needed.

What changed? In the 1950s, the standard American dinner plate was about 9 inches wide. Today, it's not uncommon to see 11–13 inch plates—a 40–60% increase in surface area. Larger plates make normal portions look puny, subconsciously encouraging us to serve (and eat) more.

And it's not just plates—it's portions across the board.

⚠ Portion Distortion Flashback:

In the 1950s, a McDonald's hamburger meal came with a 3.7-ounce burger, a 2.4-ounce serving of fries, and a 7-ounce soda.

Today's "kids' meal" offer often mirrors that same portion!

A modern combo meal? It includes a 6-8 ounce burger, 5–6 ounces of fries, and a 32-ounce drink— nearly triple the calories.

This shift in "normal" has quietly changed how we see—and consume—food. We're not necessarily more indulgent. We're just more conditioned.

Training Your Eyes to See "Enough"

It's not about deprivation. It's about recalibration.

Try these subtle swaps to help retrain your perception:

- Use salad plates instead of dinner plates for meals.

- Choose smaller bowls for things like yogurt, soup, or snacks.

- Sip from tall, narrow glasses rather than wide ones to reduce subconscious overpouring.

- Use measuring cups or pre-portioned containers when retraining.

- Eat meals without the container or packaging present—this helps your brain rely on internal cues, not branding.

Once you start seeing your plate differently, your body starts responding differently too. This isn't about tricks—it's about undoing decades of visual misinformation.

Your brain is trainable. The fork just needs a better coach.

Dining Out: Gear Up for Success

Restaurant meals can be a portion distortion minefield. In the U.S., you are almost **promised** to be overserved. Here are some strategies to navigate this challenge.

- Check the menu online for options that work for you, not against you.

- Consider splitting the entrée with a friend or opting for an appetizer as your main course.

- Request any sauces or dressings on the side.

- Ask for a to-go box right away. This way, you can enjoy a controlled portion and save the rest for another meal.

Beware of Hidden Bombs

Some of the biggest contributors to portion distortion are the invisible extras:

- Sugary drinks and specialty coffees: even a "medium" can pack more empty calories than a full meal —especially with whipped cream, syrups, or sweetened milk.

- Creamy salad dressings or added cheese

- Bread baskets or chip bowls before your meal.

These can add **hundreds of calories** without adding *true* nourishment or satisfaction.

Final Thought: Small Choices, Big Power

Your daily food choices are like pawns—easy to overlook, but capable of changing everything when used with strategy.

♟ Strategic Move #4: Balance Your Board with Real Food

- Keep a food scale on hand for recalibration weeks
- Use pre-portioned containers for busy days
- Choose smaller plates and bowls to support satiety
- Stack your plate with vegetables, not starchy sides
- Hydrate between meals to reduce false hunger cues
- Plan to take half your restaurant meal "to go".
- Pause halfway through a meal to assess fullness

You're not on a diet. You're training for *transformation*. And every portion, every plate, every pause—moves you one step closer to the win.

PLAY #5: MASTER THE CLOCK

In chess and in health, timing changes the game.

Just as a chess player must manage the ticking clock while plotting their next move, your metabolism is deeply affected by **when** you eat—not just what you eat. When time becomes your ally, the entire board shifts in your favor.

This chapter introduces one of the most powerful strategies in the weight loss game: **Intermittent Fasting (IF)**. By aligning your eating window with your body's natural rhythms, you can unlock deeper metabolic healing, improve insulin sensitivity, and even reduce inflammation. Let's explore how to master your metabolic clock.

The Science Behind Intermittent Fasting

Intermittent fasting involves cycling between periods of eating and fasting, rather than following the traditional "three meals a day" approach. During a fasted state, your body undergoes powerful metabolic shifts:

- **Insulin levels drop**, allowing the body to access fat stores for energy.

- **Fat burning increases**, supporting weight loss.

- **Autophagy (cellular cleanup)** is triggered, helping your body recycle damaged cells.

- **Inflammation may decrease**, improving long-term health outcomes.

But this is not just a trendy diet—it's a return to our biological roots. For most of human history, fasting wasn't a choice. It was normal. Our ancestors went hours, even days, between meals depending on availability.

Today, our constant snacking culture keeps insulin high and metabolism sluggish.

But there's another layer: **your circadian rhythm.** Your body's internal clock regulates hormone release—like insulin, cortisol, and melatonin—based on light and dark cycles. Eating late at night can confuse this system, elevating blood sugar, disrupting sleep, and triggering fat storage.

Simply put: **Your body expects food when the sun is up.** Aligning your eating window with daylight hours can enhance hormonal harmony and improve your weight loss results.

A Reality Check

I once had a patient—a minister—who completed a 40-day "biblical" fast, drinking only water. **And yet... she lost no weight.** It was a wake-up call: **calories aren't the only factor.** Timing, hormones, sleep, stress, and overall metabolic flexibility all matter.

So when people say, "But isn't breakfast the most important meal of the day?"—my answer is: it depends.

If you do physical labor or have high energy demands early in the day, yes—fueling in the morning makes sense. But for many people with more sedentary schedules, waiting until later to eat can work better with their hormones and metabolism.

Exploring Different Fasting Schedules:

Not all fasting is created equal. Here are the most common approaches:

- **16/8 Method**: Fast for 16 hours, eat during an 8-hour window (e.g., 12–8 p.m.).

- **5:2 Method**: Eat normally 5 days per week; restrict calories to 500–600 for 2 non-consecutive days.

- **Eat Stop Eat**: 24-hour fasts once or twice per week.

I most often recommend the **16/8** structure, starting with something like an 11 a.m.–7 p.m. window. During the morning, stick with water, black coffee, or unsweetened tea to stay hydrated and support your fast.

→ *Note: If you take medications or have metabolic conditions (like diabetes or get "hangry" if you don't eat), consult your provider first. Fasting isn't one-size-fits-all.*

Play the Clock on and off the Board

In chess, the Knight doesn't move in a straight line, and neither does lasting weight loss. To win, you'll need smart timing, strategic angles, and a few moves that may feel unfamiliar at first.

Weight loss isn't just about *when* you eat—it's also about how well your body recovers between moves. Timing your meals is powerful... but timing your rest, connection, and restoration? That's the long-game mastery most people miss.

Here are two crucial—but often overlooked—factors that influence your weight more than you realize:

1. **Sleep** like your progress depends on it—because it does.

   - Poor sleep raises cortisol and ghrelin, making you hungrier and more prone to stress-eating.

   - Leptin, your fullness hormone, drops—leaving you chasing satisfaction all day.

     - **Aim for 7–9 hours of consistent, quality sleep.** This is non-negotiable. Rest is when your body repairs, regulates hormones, and resets metabolism.

     - **Bonus advantage:** Sleeping in sync with daylight supports your circadian rhythm, improves energy, and makes intermittent fasting more effective. As the saying goes, "Early to bed, early to rise…" isn't just poetic—it's *strategic*.

     - **Night shift or swing shift?** You're playing the game on hard mode. Our biology wasn't designed to thrive when working at night. While it may not be realistic to change your schedule immediately, prioritize restoring a natural rhythm whenever possible.

2. **The power of connection and pleasure.**

- Physical affection and intimacy (in any form that feels right for you) reduces stress, and supports healthy hormone regulation.

- Sexual activity can burn about 70-100kcal per session.

- When we feel safe and connected, we're less likely to reach for food to soothe loneliness, boredom, or shame.

- This isn't about performance—it's about presence. Give yourself permission to *enjoy your body now*, not just when you reach your goal. Loving yourself along the way isn't always easy—but it is a winning strategy.

Final Thought: Time is Your Secret Weapon

You don't need another meal plan—you need a **metabolic rhythm**.

When you master the clock, you reduce inflammation, retrain insulin naturally, and create space for your body to heal. Just like in chess, mastering the middle game of time can set you up for a winning endgame.

♟ Strategic Move #5: Move Like a Knight

Master the art of timing your moves—fasting, sleeping, even intimacy—for metabolic advantage.

- Start with a 12-hour fast and gradually work toward 14–16 hours

- Keep your eating window consistent (e.g., 11 a.m.–7 p.m.)

- Only eat when it's daylight out (syncs with circadian rhythm)

- Stay hydrated in the morning: water, black coffee (decaf is even better), unsweetened herbal teas

- Break your fast with a balanced meal rich in protein, fiber, and healthy fat

- Use apps or timers to track your eating windows for accountability

- Whenever possible, align your eating hours with daylight to support hormonal health

- Sleep! Best is by 10 PM. Use blackout curtains, avoid screens 30-60 minutes before your "bedtime".

- Create connections—Light a candle. Initiate a meaningful hug. Physical intimacy helps regulate hormones, improves mood, and yes—can burn a few bonus calories too.

PLAY #6: ACTIVATE YOUR PIECES

*"You can't win a game of chess with your
pieces stuck on the back row."*

Ever tried working out, maybe even with a trainer, but the scale just doesn't budge? Yes, muscle weighs more than fat, but it also burns more fuel than fat, so after a while, the scale should "reward" you, right?

The truth is, most weight loss begins in the mouth—not the gym.

I've worked with countless gym-goers and even gym owners who couldn't shed those last stubborn pounds.

Why? Because movement is powerful, but it's not the main driver of weight loss. Still, in the long game of health and long-term vitality, movement plays a critical role. And like chess, you can't expect progress if you never move your pieces.

While it's absolutely possible to lose weight without exercise—and many of our clients do—*keeping* that weight off, protecting muscle, and feeling good in your body for the long haul? That's where strategic movement comes in.

This chapter is about **activating your body strategically**—not with punishment, but with purpose. Let's explore how movement reduces inflammation, protects muscle, and supports a healthy metabolism—without becoming a slave to the gym.

Why Movement Matters (Even If You're Not a "Gym Person")

Our increasingly sedentary lifestyles have changed what our bodies need. We now spend most of our days sitting—at desks, in cars, on couches. Compare that to a few generations ago. My great-grandfather started farming with a horse and plow. Even housework required real muscle. We've gone from physically engaged to technology tethered.

The problem? When you lose weight **without movement**, you often lose muscle, too. That makes future weight regain more likely and increases the risk of falls, fatigue, and frailty. The old saying is true: **"Move it or lose it."**

People often ask how to lose weight and *keep* muscle. When I explain that keeping muscle means *using* it, I sometimes see resistance in their face. But think of a broken arm in a cast. When the cast comes off, that arm is visibly smaller and weaker. Only by *using* the muscle again does it regain its strength and shape. Your entire body is no different.

But here's the kicker—it doesn't have to be complicated or even very time consuming and you don't need a gym membership to activate your body's full potential.

You cannot out-work a bad diet, though. Weight loss is more about what you have in your hand when you do that bicep curl to your mouth. But for longevity and wellness, keeping active has been shown to not only protect your muscle, but your brain and memory, too.

Stay in the Game with Strength

Cardio helps your heart and endurance—but to keep muscle, you have to use it. Resistance training doesn't require a gym.

Even if you knew George Foreman primarily as the face behind the famous countertop grill, you might not have realized his bigger legacy. He was a two-time heavyweight boxing champion who shocked the world by reclaiming his title *in his 40s*—using nothing more than bodyweight exercises to rebuild his fitness.

His comeback wasn't powered by fancy machines—it was fueled by strategic, consistent movement. Like activating overlooked chess pieces, he proved that no matter your age or starting point, **your body can do more than you think**—when you start moving with intention.

- **Try resistance bands, light weights, or your own body.** Squats, wall push-ups, planks, and lunges can all provide powerful results without costing a dime or requiring a gym pass.
- **Consistency over intensity**. 20–30 minutes, 3 times per week, is a great place to start.

♟ **Pro Tip:** Want my go-to home-friendly resistance + cardio combo? My family and I personally use a program that blends low-impact cardio with functional strength movements—perfect for beginners or those getting back into a routine. It supports fat loss, reduces stress, protects lean muscle, and is designed to be joint-friendly and time-efficient.

While I didn't create the program myself, I wholeheartedly recommend it because it meets you where you are—with scalable options for all fitness levels. Whether you're just starting or picking things back up, it's a proven framework for getting results without a gym.

♟ Email hello@RootCauseRewire.com with subject line: MOVEMENT and we'll send you the details.

The Inflammation Connection

Balanced, consistent movement helps naturally reduce inflammation, that fire that spreads and leads to many chronic health issues. Here's how:

- **Boosts Anti-Inflammatory Myokines**: These healing compounds are released during exercise and help fight inflammation.
- **Improves Circulation**: Movement delivers nutrients and oxygen while flushing waste from tissues. It also strengthens the heart— your most vital muscle—which beats more than 100,000 times a day to keep you alive. Regular movement helps that rhythm stay strong and steady.
- **Lowers Cortisol**: Exercise done right lowers stress hormones and increases feel-good brain chemicals.

♟ **Note for Night Shift Workers**: If you work swing shifts or overnights, your hormones can get out of sync, making fat loss and energy regulation more challenging. Strategic movement—especially during your "wake window"—can help rebalance cortisol, reduce inflammation, and keep your metabolism responsive. Even short walks or bodyweight movement during your shift break can make a difference.

But more isn't always better.

When Exercise Backfires

Some people hit the gym hard….and still see the scale stall. Here's why:

1. **The Reward Trap:** You had a great workout or did a lot more activity than normal and "deserve" a reward, so you indulge in a bigger meal or in your not-so-healthy beverage…instantly undoing your workout benefits.

2. **Overtraining Stress**: Intense workouts can actually raise cortisol—your stress hormone—tricking your body into survival mode, as if you're constantly 'running from a bear.' In this mode, the body clings to energy reserves,

often storing fat (especially belly fat) as a backup. It's a paradox—more effort can lead to more storage. Like in chess, overextending your pieces without a solid strategy can leave you vulnerable and stuck.

If you're doing everything "right" and still not seeing results, it may be time to dial back the intensity.

♟ Pro tip: If you can hold a conversation while you work out, you're staying in the sweet spot for fat burning and inflammation reduction.

Start Where You Are

Don't let the search for the "perfect" workout stall your progress. Your job isn't to win the fitness Olympics—it's to **activate your pieces** and stay in the game.

- **Walking**: Underrated, always available, and powerful. Aim to go a little farther each day—and when possible, take paths with some hills to keep challenging your body and building heart strength.

- **Dancing, Yoga, Biking, Pilates**: All count. Choose what you enjoy.

- **Resistance counts too**—and now you know why.

No excuses—escape the "Nation of Procrasta"! With all the free resources online at your fingertips, you can find beginner or hotel-style workouts that match your time, tempo, and taste.

By embracing movement, you'll strengthen your body and cultivate a calmer and more resilient mind.

Accountability Is a Game-Changer

You don't have to go it alone. Having an accountability partner—or better yet, a team—can double your chances of success. Cravings and setbacks are inevitable. But with support, you're less likely to quit.

Sometimes, your current circle may not fully support or understand your goals. Whether it's subtle sabotage or simply a lack of shared vision, **it's okay** to seek out new allies.

Find people who are already doing what you aspire to do—whether that's prioritizing healthy meals, making time to move, or simply speaking more positively about their bodies. Ask one or two of them to hold you accountable, cheer you on, or check in weekly. It can make all the difference.

♟ **Pro Tip**: Build a group of 3. That way, someone's always available even if one person can't show up.

In our programs, we include weekly check-ins and a private online community because we know: **consistency beats intensity every time.**

♟ **Permission Granted**: You don't need to "deserve" support to seek it out. If you do better with structure—use it. If a gym membership, a class pass, or a group coaching program helps you follow through, there is no shame in that. In fact, for many, having something on the calendar or someone expecting you to show up is exactly the thing that shifts the mindset from "maybe I'll try" to "this is who I am now."

Structure isn't a crutch—it's scaffolding for your success. Think of it as an act of self-respect, not self-doubt.

The best plan isn't the hardest one—it's the one you'll actually follow, especially when life gets busy. Whether you're showing up for yourself, a group, or a coach, what matters most is that you keep showing up. One move at a time.

Final Thought: Don't Keep Your Power on the Sidelines

In chess, the strongest pieces can't help you if they're stuck in place. Your body is no different. When you activate your muscles, you're not just building strength—you're protecting your progress.

♟ Strategic Move #6: Activate Your Pieces

- Choose **movement you enjoy** to make it sustainable.
- Aim for **20–30 minutes of moderate activity**, 3+ days a week.
- Mix in **resistance training** to protect your muscle and metabolism.
- **Track your movement** and celebrate consistency, not perfection.
- Get **accountability support**—in person or online.
- Need inspiration?

♟ Email hello@RootCauseRewire.com with subject line: MOVEMENT and we'll send you the details on the program we personally use and clients have loved.

CHECK-IN: POWER UP YOUR PIECES

You can't out-train a bad eating plan, but if you don't *move it*, you *lose it*—especially when it comes to your muscle, energy, and long-term results.

🎯 **Time to assess your position on the board:**

- Where are you at today, physically and emotionally?

- Where do you want to be—90 days from now? One year from now?

- How much time are you actually moving your body each week?

- How far could you walk without being winded?

- What areas of your body are you most concerned about or want to strengthen?

- What small moves can you start making to get momentum on your side?

- Who are three people who could support or encourage you on this journey?

- And most importantly… are you keeping your strongest "pieces" in play—or leaving them stuck on the sidelines?

Strength isn't about going harder—it's about consistent, strategic positioning. Movement stabilizes your emotional board and empowers you to hold your ground.

PLAY #7: THE CHECKMATE MOVE

The most powerful piece on the board?
Your emotional state. Emotional sabotage
can unravel even the most well-planned
strategies. Learn to protect your inner
Queen.

Our weight journey isn't just about movement and meals. This play dives into your most powerful tool: your mind.

We all start strong—but what helps us *finish*? It's not just willpower or grit. It's the ability to recognize old patterns, release what's not working, and lead yourself with vision and compassion. This is how you win the long game.

The Gremlins on the Board: Self-Sabotage Unveiled

You've felt it. That voice that whispers: "You've already blown it." "You're not cut out for this." "Start over on Monday."

Those are mental saboteurs—what I call your **gremlins**. They hijack your progress, not because you're weak—but because your nervous system is trying to *protect* you.

Common ways they show up:

- **All-or-Nothing Thinking**: One slip turns into total derailment.

- **Negative Self-Talk**: You berate yourself for small mistakes.

- **Emotional Eating**: Food becomes comfort instead of fuel.

- **The Knowing/Doing Gap**: "I know what to do… I just don't do it." That's your inner gremlin speaking.

Conditioned Behaviors: The Real Programming

Our past experiences and societal influences can shape our present behaviors. It is now thought that by age 10, your emotional blueprint is largely formed. The way you respond to food, stress, praise, punishment—it's learned. Passed down. And often, outdated—kept alive by emotional ties, unspoken fears, or simply repetition. But you're not locked in. Awareness gives you the upper hand—and permission to play a new move.

Your body has been keeping the score—based on past experiences, comments, and emotions tied to food or your physical self. One woman I worked with shared how she always cleaned her plate—not because she was hungry, but because her mother praised her for being a "good girl" when she did. Another client realized she unconsciously avoided eating healthy because it reminded her of the restrictive, shame-filled diets her father put her on in high school.

These experiences may seem small—but to your emotional brain, they were defining. And that part of your brain? It doesn't operate in years. It lives in moments.

Your mind really doesn't know the concept of time. Have you ever heard a song on the radio and mentally taken right back to high school? Or have you had a smell transport you back to Grandma's house? Then you've experienced this yourself!

- Were you told to clean your plate?

- Did food = love in your family?

- Did you absorb shame from early teasing or criticism?

- Were desserts or snacks used as a reward—or withheld as punishment?

- Was your body shape or size criticized—even casually?

- Do you still feel you have to "earn" your food or justify eating something you enjoy?

Your brain stores these moments. And your nervous system tries to keep you "safe" by repeating them—no matter how illogical it seems now.

Good news? You can rewrite the script.

And if you've struggled to keep weight off, **there's a good chance emotional eating has been your body's way of coping** with stress, pressure, or unmet needs.

You're not broken. You're just patterned.

Emotional Eating: Your #1 Opponent

If you're like most women I work with, stress eating isn't just a bad habit—it's a survival mechanism. When life gets hard, your body wants comfort. Fast. Familiar. So it turns to food.

That's not failure. That's a nervous system in overdrive, doing what it was trained to do.

But here's the truth: You don't need to shame yourself.
You just need to understand your patterns—and rewire them.

One woman I worked with came in wanting to lose weight. And yet, after every bit of progress, she stalled. Through our work, she uncovered something she hadn't admitted—not even to herself. Deep down, she didn't want to lose the weight. Why? Because if she did, her husband might want to be intimate again. And she wasn't emotionally ready for that. Her weight had become a form of protection.

Another client ate perfectly all week—until stress hit. Then it was fast food, sugar, and guilt. Not because she didn't know better, but because stress short-circuited her system. Sound familiar?

You're not alone. And you're not the problem.

Building a Growth Mindset

If you want lasting change, you must lead your mind like a master player leads the board. That means:

- **Challenge Negative Thoughts**: Name the gremlin. Replace the script. "I've failed before" becomes "I'm learning to succeed now."

- **Play the Long Game**: Weight loss is a journey. Progress beats perfection. Track wins, not just losses.

- **Train Your Inner Voice**: Talk to yourself like a friend you're coaching with love. That voice becomes your internal compass. Your words matter.

Growth isn't about doing more. It's about **thinking differently**—so your habits can finally follow.

Strengthen the Mental Game: Deep Dive

Want to go deeper? Over the last several years, I've helped hundreds of clients identify and neutralize their gremlins using a proven, body-guided approach—not therapy, not talk, but hands-on rewiring.

It's powerful. It's gentle. And it works—even when you don't know where to start.

We've worked through:

- **Hidden fears about being seen or desired**
- **Beliefs that success = danger**
- **Food memories linked to trauma, safety, or comfort**
- **Guilt, shame, and "deservedness" blocks**

Sometimes it's small. Sometimes it's huge. But every breakthrough brings clarity—and often, momentum.

One thing I love about this process? It doesn't require you to *talk it all out.* It's not therapy—though it can complement therapy beautifully. It's a nervous system reset, using simple but profound tools rooted in neuroscience and energy medicine.

Through this technique, I've helped clients dissolve long-held shame, uncover the real roots of stress eating, and finally feel safe in their skin— without relying on talk therapy or needing to "figure it all out" first.

While I love this work—and it's truly been life-changing for many I've helped—the reality is, there's only one of me. I can only take on so many clients at a time. I hate turning people away or knowing that someone desperately needs this kind of breakthrough, yet doesn't have the time, ability, or means to travel for in-person sessions.

That's exactly why I created an online course: to make DIY-friendly versions of these powerful tools available without barriers. Your healing shouldn't depend on geography, time off work, or waiting for a spot to open up. You deserve support when you're ready—on your own terms.

Rewire Emotional Eating: Master the Mind, Transform the Body is a guided 6-week experience that brings the same mind-body principles I use with clients in my office directly to you. It's flexible, practical, and designed to support deep transformation without disrupting your life.

No travel. No waitlist. Just powerful tools you can start using now to finally shift the patterns behind stress eating and self-sabotage.

♟ Strategic Move #7: Unlock the Hidden Power

Your greatest transformation starts in your mind. After thousands of client sessions, I've discovered 4 core emotional eating types — each driven by different subconscious "Pawn State" patterns.

Take the quiz to uncover your unique type and receive a powerful bonus that shows you how to transform self-sabotage into strategy — moving from Pawn survival into your Queen state of freedom, flexibility, and sovereignty.

Take the quiz and claim your gift: visit https://quiz.rewireemotionaleating.com or scan the QR code and discover your type. Use the code **CHECKMATE** to get your personalized guide completely free (a $29 value)—your first step in breaking the cycle for good.

You now have more than one powerful way to work with me to Rewire Emotional Eating:

- The 6-week course: **Master the Mind, Transform the Body**—a self-paced, guided experience built to transform your inner game.

- Or, when ready, apply for **in-person breakthrough sessions** or future **retreats** for live, hands-on support.

Whatever path you choose, just know: your next move could be the one that finally frees you.

This is your Checkmate moment—and I'd love to personally help you make it a win.

SELF-CHECK: YOUR INNER OPPONENT

Let's take a mini-course approach to challenging negative thoughts and promoting growth.

Take a moment to be still and reflect.

When it comes to losing weight, what messages come to mind?

Write them down without censoring yourself.

Now pause and ask: where might each of those messages have come from?

> Your mom? A doctor? Your grandma making comments about your mother's weight? A coach, classmate, or social media influence?

There's no right or wrong answers.

Sometimes just naming the source helps loosen the grip that message has held over you.

Next, rewrite each message into a more empowering belief.

For example: "I've been overweight my whole life, so why bother now?"

Becomes: "I've been overweight until now—but I'm learning new ways to care for my body and release what I no longer need."

Use language that feels authentic to you. The more it sounds like *your* voice, the more powerful it becomes.

Once you've written your new statements, post them somewhere visible.

Read them daily—especially aloud, in the mirror if possible.

That way, your brain **hears and sees you** becoming the person you're growing into:

- your handwriting (especially if in cursive),
- your eyes reading it,
- your voice speaking it,
- your ears and mind hearing it,
- and you, seeing yourself in the mirror as you say it....

This is a **masterful** play with powerful results.

Want more? Join the Rewire Emotional Eating: Master the Mind, Transform the Body course.

CLAIM YOUR VICTORY

"Your final moves matter most."

We've covered a lot of ground together—more than most traditional weight loss programs ever touch. From inflammation and food sensitivities to toxins, fasting, movement, and mindset, you now hold a complete picture of what it really takes to transform—not just lose weight, but *heal* from the inside out.

How many of these elements were part of your strategy before this book? If your answer is "not many," you're not alone. That's exactly why I created this strategic guide.

After working with thousands of clients, I'm more convinced than ever that sustainable weight loss requires a *whole-person* approach—not another gimmick, shot, or short-term fix.

Introducing Root Cause Rewire: Weight Reset System™

Our 9-week weight loss-focused program—**Root Cause Rewire: Weight Reset System™**—was built on the very principles you've just read, rooted in my Root Cause Rewire approach and S-T-S Method: Sensitivities – Toxins – Stress.

It's not a diet. It's a system of realignment: resetting your metabolism, calming inflammation, and rewiring the hidden drivers of self-sabotage.

And it works. Most clients lose 20–40 pounds in 9 weeks while experiencing:

- **No hunger**
- **No shots or weight loss pills**
- **No prepackaged meals**
- **No calorie counting or point tracking**

Why? Because those things don't lead to lasting change—and let's be honest, they aren't enjoyable or sustainable either.

Instead, our clients experience real results through:

Whole-food nutrition that calms inflammation
Elimination of toxic triggers
Loss of "gremlins" or bad mental programming
Customization through targeted testing
Healing from the inside out—body, mind, and metabolism

More Than Just Weight Loss

When the root causes are rewired, inflammation is reduced and the body is supported properly, amazing things happen.

Many clients report:

✓ Deeper sleep

✓ Better energy and mood

✓ Better self image and libido

✓ Less pain and stiffness

✓ Reduced blood pressure or cholesterol

✓ Healthier blood sugar levels

✓ Decreased medications (with physician approval)

✓ Greater self-trust, confidence, and clarity

We've been honored to be voted *Best Weight Loss Program* in our area multiple years in a row—and the real credit goes to our clients, who dared to try a new path and stuck with it.

If you're ready to activate your own transformation with a system and approach that embraces all of the Masterplan moves, we'd love to walk beside you.

Final Thought:

Your transformation isn't just about the scale—It's emotional. It's neurological. It's deeply personal.

Whether you join **Root Cause Rewire: Weight Reset System**™ to make every Masterplan move…

Or begin applying these strategies on your own…

The most powerful move on the board… is still yours to make.

♟ Your Final Strategic Move: Own the Game

Whether this book has sparked your first "a-ha" moment—or you've already taken bold steps like completing your food sensitivity test or beginning the *Rewire Emotional Eating: Master the Mind, Transform the Body*™ journey—you're not done yet.

Your next move? Choose the path that best fits your strategy:

- **Food Testing:** Visit **foods2lose.com** to uncover hidden food triggers and receive my personal Loom follow-up.

- **Quiz & Queen Guide:** Discover your emotional eating type and use the code **CHECKMATE** to unlock your $29 Queen Guide free.

- **The Winning Program:** Step into the **Root Cause Rewire™ — Weight Reset System**, the all-inclusive reset you've just read about, designed to bring every piece of the STS method together for lasting transformation. Learn more and reserve your spot at **www.RootCauseRewire.com/weight**

*Every move you make from here is a chance
to claim your power back. The only
question is—will you take it?*

Real Results from Clients

"I lost 30 pounds doing the 9-week program. I have since lost another 25 pounds, and I still follow what I learned in the program. I love it!" — Cathy A.

"I was able to lose almost a pound a day without extreme exercise. I learned many positive health habits and even learned I actually do like vegetables!"— Dennis H.

"I loved the whole program. I finally stopped obsessing about food. For the first time, I feel calm around eating— and in control. I haven't been this size since college." — Jackie R.

"I thought I was doing all the "right" things and eating healthy, but the food testing revealed many of the things I was eating were not good for me. With Dr. Welch's help, I discovered simple shifts that made all the difference... I feel like a new man.!."— Trevor N.

"Dr. Welch's program was truly amazing. If more people knew about it, it would be a complete game changer in the weight loss field. The whole picture—the process— was exactly what I needed. I truly feel like a different person after going through it. Thank you, Dr. Welch." —Ashley M.

"I was skeptical after trying many approaches, but this program was a game-changer for me. I lost over 50 pounds in just 2 months and have kept it off for over two and a half years now by continuing to use what I learned from Dr. Welch and her team."—*Jeff B.*

"I didn't even realize I had been using food to feel safe until we did this work. Rewiring that part of me—that shift changed everything for me—not just the number on the scale."—*Julie R.*

"I highly recommend the Root Cause Rewire program. *As with any weight loss program, you have to be ready to do what YOU need to do in order to be successful. The program is easy to follow, and the support and accountability are there if you need it, which I did. I lost 40 pounds in 9 weeks and have kept it off. It's a great program."*— *Becky G.*

> *"When people reflect on their lives, it's not*
> *the mistakes we regret most —*
> *it's the chances we didn't take,*
> *the changes we avoided,*
> *and the courage we never claimed."*
> *— Dr. Jennifer Welch*

ABOUT THE AUTHOR

Dr. Jennifer Welch is a functional health expert and Doctor of Chiropractic with a lifelong passion for natural healing. Even as a child, she questioned the overuse of medications, instinctively drawn to more holistic ways of supporting the body. That passion eventually became her profession.

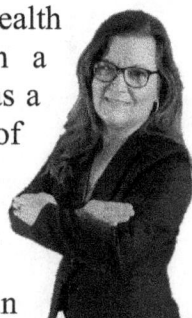

Since opening her private practice in 2008, Dr. Welch has helped thousands reclaim their health—naturally. From stubborn weight struggles to chronic conditions that conventional care couldn't resolve, her approach blends clinical precision with compassionate care.

With advanced certifications in **nutrition, neurology, and neuro-emotional health**, she invests hundreds of hours annually in continuing education to stay at the forefront of integrative medicine. Her mission is clear: **To help people heal faster, more deeply, and with the fewest interventions possible.**

Her signature weight loss program, **Root Cause Rewire: Weight Reset System™**, is a strategic, science-backed program based on her foundational S-T-S Method™ framework. Clients lose weight, reduce inflammation, and reclaim confidence by addressing not just diet—but detox, emotional patterns, and metabolic resistance.

Whether guiding clients through her Root Cause Rewire Systems, teaching emotional eating breakthroughs, or speaking on national stages, Dr. Welch helps people reconnect with their bodies, reset their biology, and create lasting change—without fads, extremes, or shame.

www.ingramcontent.com/pod-product-compliance
Lightning Source LLC
Chambersburg PA
CBHW070812280326
41934CB00012B/3165